KT-238-402

Overcoming Common Problems

Dr Dawn's Guide to Toddler Health

DR DAWN HARPER

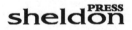
sheldon PRESS

First published in Great Britain in 2016

Sheldon Press
36 Causton Street
London SW1P 4ST
www.sheldonpress.co.uk

British Library Cataloguing-in-Publication Data
A catalogue record for this book is available from the British Library

ISBN 978–1–84709–393–6
eBook ISBN 978–1–84709–398–1

Typeset by Fakenham Prepress Solutions, Fakenham, Norfolk NR21 8NN
First printed in Great Britain by Ashford Colour Press
Subsequently digitally reprinted in Great Britain

eBook by Fakenham Prepress Solutions, Fakenham, Norfolk NR21 8NN

Produced on paper from sustainable forests

To my three lovely children,
Charlie, Eleanor and Harvey.
Thank you for all the fond memories

Contents

Introduction

This book is designed to follow on from *Dr Dawn's Guide to Your Baby's First Year*, and in it I hope to guide you through the amazing changes that you will notice in the next three years.

I will try to cover everything from teething and feeding to sleeping, and the developmental milestones you can expect to see. I will also cover the ailments that can afflict our toddlers and give advice on what you can do to look after them and when you really should see a doctor. I will explain the vaccination schedule and the illnesses they protect against, and what you should have in your medicine cabinet along with a simple guide to first aid tips that you should know.

But, before I start let me give you one piece of advice. I'm not speaking as a doctor now, I am speaking as a parent to other parents. In the next three years, your son or daughter will do things and say things that are so heart-warming you think you will burst with love for them and some will make you laugh so much you cry. These things are so amazing at the time that you think you will remember them forever. Some of them you will, but many you will forget, so my advice to you is to invest in a hardback notebook and whenever one of those episodes occurs, jot it down. That book will become one of your most treasured possessions in years to come and ultimately will be enjoyed by your children when they are adults, and even by their children. I know when my kids were small they loved nothing more than to hear stories from my mum about the things I got up to as a kid, and keeping a notebook like this will give you so much more material!

1

Developmental checks and milestones

Every child who is registered with an NHS GP will be called for regular reviews. It is important that you attend these as if there are any issues with your child's development, this is when they are likely to be picked up. And, if any problems are discovered, the earlier we can put systems into place to help a child who is lagging behind in his or her development the better the outlook. You can of course talk to your health visitor or GP at any time between these appointments if you have concerns.

Routine checks

12 months

A general health check is done at one year old. This is an opportunity to discuss any concerns that you have. The health care professional in charge of the clinic will want to do a full overview of your child's development, including speech and language skills, physical development and growth, and diet and behaviour.

2–2.5 years

This is your child's third full health review and will cover everything from growth, behaviour, sleep, diet and teething to general health and any concerns that you may have.

4–5 years

This is what we used to call the pre-school medical. Your child will be weighed and measured and these measurements are plotted on graphs to check that your child is growing appropriately. Your child's vision and hearing will be checked and all aspects of his or her general development will be discussed.

Milestones

The following is simply a guideline. As I have said many times before, children are as individual as we are as adults and they will vary in the way in which they develop. This is simply to give you an idea of the sort of time frame in which you can expect your child to achieve certain milestones. If your child was born prematurely, we allow for that up until the age of two. What I mean by that is that if your baby was born a month prematurely, your child may take an extra month to reach each milestone, but after the age of two we would expect your child to have caught up with his or her peers and develop at the same rate as them.

12 months

By the time your baby is a year old he or she should be able to let go of objects or hand them to someone on request. Your child will recognize shapes and will start to be able to put through shapes in matching holes. Playing with toys that encourage this will aid this development and calling the shapes by name as you do this will help your child's speech and language development.

From 10 to 18 months

This is the time when you can expect your child to start walking independently. Your child will, of course, be a little precarious at first and will fall often but if he or she is not showing any signs of walking independently by 18 months, it is worth talking to your health visitor.

11–12 months

Your child should start to be enjoying feeding him- or herself with finger food. This will prove very messy to start and it is much quicker and easier to continue to feed him or her, but go with it. This is an important part of development. Don't ever leave your child unattended with food at this stage, though, as there is a risk of choking.

12 months

Your child should recognize his or her name by now and turn toward you if you call it. He or she will also be able to grasp the concept that an object still exists even when it is removed from vision so will enjoy games like 'peek-a-boo'. I remember we nick-named my first child 'where's-e-gone' at about this stage as he would walk around repeating that phrase again and again!

From 12 to 18 months

At this stage your child will be starting to gain a vocabulary. Your child may have as many as 20 recognizable words and will rec-ognize many more so will be able to point to objects on request. Reading to your child regularly at this stage and talking to him or her will help to expand this.

13–15 months

This is when your child may start to show a degree of independ-ence. Your child may want to remove clothes – shoes and socks are the specialty here and it can be frustrating but it is your child's way of becoming his or her own person and you will get very good at replacing them! Your child will also be ready to expand his or her diet by trying new foods and textures. Your child may refuse some at first. Don't make a big deal of it, just offer the food again at another point.

15–18 months

Around now, your child may enjoy building towers of bricks. Encourage your child with this and try to make time every day to play this game and praise his or her achievement. Your child will respond well to your enthusiasm and want to do more.

18 months – 2 years

Your child will begin to be able to kick or throw a ball by now and should be able to string two words together and point to parts of his or her own body.

1.5–4 years

Children vary hugely in when they develop bladder control and are ready for potty training (see Chapter 5) and it can happen at any time during this window.

1.5–5 years

During this period your child will start to enjoy colouring and painting. This can be a particularly messy time but it is an important developmental milestone and should be encouraged. Your child's portraits of you will bear no resemblance to the human form to begin with, but always show delight and encouragement and your child will thrive on this. You can also point out colours to your child so that he or she starts to understand the concept of colour.

3–4 years

This is the time when your child may start nursery. All children under 5 are entitled to a minimum of 12.5 hours of free nursery education for 38 weeks of the year. Your child may be reluctant at first. I remember my daughter, in particular, was very clingy when I took her to nursery and I found it really hard to leave her. It feels dreadful and all you want to do is to take them back home, but if you stand out of view and observe for a while you will see how quickly most children just get on with it as soon as you are out of sight, meaning you can get on with your day without feeling like the parent from hell. Socializing is an important part of a child's development.

At this stage your child should also be talking in short sentences and be able to sing nursery rhymes – something that will be encouraged in a nursery environment too. Your child's pictures should become more recognizable as what they are supposed to be too! Your child will enjoy television and this will give you a good opportunity to get some of your chores done, but be careful – your child will also need input and encouragement from you and too much time in front of a screen will not provide him or her with the stimulation needed. I recommend limiting any TV watching to a maximum of two hours a day.

2

Feeding and nutrition

By the age of 18 months your child should be eating pretty much the kind of foods that you do but, of course, your child's meals will be significantly smaller – probably about a third to a half the size of yours. As a rough guide, toddlers need between 1,000 and 1,400 calories a day depending on their size and level of activity. Your child will need protein at every meal and you will notice that during growth spurts, and certainly when your child starts walking, his or her appetite will increase. Go with this and don't be worried about giving snacks between meals. If you can, try to avoid high-sugar snacks and opt for healthy snacks such as raw fruit and vegetables. Your child will need food from every food group – fats, proteins, fruit and vegetables and carbohydrates, and the more variety you can introduce the better. It's a good idea to allow your child to sit at the table in a high chair and eat with you as a family. It may be a messy affair and not the most relaxing to begin with, but will get your child into the habit of eating and socializing at mealtimes as a family.

Even a varied diet is unlikely to provide a growing child with enough vitamin A, C and D so the Department of Health recommends that children under the age of five are given vitamin drops to supplement their diet. Your health visitor will advise you on which drops you need. Make sure you stick to the recommended dose as too much of some vitamins can be harmful.

Don't add salt or sugar to a toddler's food and avoid low-fat varieties in young children as they need some fat in their diet and food advertised as low-fat is often high in sugar. Avoid small pieces of food and nuts that a small child could choke on and never leave a toddler unobserved when eating finger food.

You should avoid shark, swordfish and tuna as these may contain mercury, which is harmful to the developing toddler.

You can give eggs to a child from the age of 6 months provided your child is not allergic to them, but make sure they are thoroughly cooked.

What about milk?

You may or may not be breastfeeding your toddler, but after the age of a year it is OK to introduce cow's milk. Use full-fat cow's milk at first as this contains the fat and fat soluble vitamins that your child will need for development. From the age of two, if they are thriving and growing well you can use semi-skimmed milk if you wish and after aged five, it is OK to use skimmed milk.

What about other drinks?

A baby over six months can drink tap water without the need to boil it first and water is probably the best option for your toddler to drink when he or she is thirsty.

Fruit juices are rich in vitamin C but also contain natural sugars so try to limit them to about 150 ml a day and, where possible, dilute them with water.

Try to avoid fizzy drinks if you can. They are usually high in sugar and will make your child feel full, which may mean your child doesn't eat the nutritious calories you want him or her to eat later in the day.

When can I expect my toddler to use a regular cup?

Most two year olds are capable of using a regular cup but some prefer to stick with a straw or a sippy cup and there is nothing wrong with this. Your child will eventually want to copy you and be like a grown-up so let your child do this in his or her own time.

3

Dressing

Any time from around a year old, your child may start to show an interest in dressing him- or herself. Initially, it may just be wanting to hold out a leg for you to put on socks or shoes, but gradually your child will want to do more and more without assistance.

Sadly for you, your child is likely to become adept at undressing much earlier than dressing, which can be frustrating when you are trying to get out of the house. I had three children in three years and when they were all tiny I remember thinking I would never get out of the house – no sooner was one fully dressed than another one had started to remove various layers! It is, however, an important part of development and although it can take a lot longer to allow our children to get involved with the dressing process than it ever would to just do it all ourselves, their interest is to be encouraged. Girls tend to start to want to dress themselves earlier than boys.

The best way to start is probably encouraging them to put on simple things like pyjamas. Once they have mastered this you can go on to day clothes. Make things easy for your child by placing clothes out in the order in which they need to be put on and, wherever possible, opt for easy fastenings to begin with, so poppers and Velcro rather than buttons and laces.

When your child is ready to start with buttons, try to find a garment with large buttons to make life easier. From the age of about 18 months, most toddlers enjoy dressing up so this might be the perfect opportunity to introduce buttons.

By about two or three your child will probably be able to tackle zips but tying shoe laces will come a lot later.

Toddlers grow at a rapid rate and dressing them can be an expensive hobby as they are likely to grow out of clothes rather than wear them out – it is worth bearing that in mind when you are shopping.

Toddlers' feet will change quickly too and you may have to have your child's feet remeasured as frequently as every two to three months during growth spurts.

4

Bathing and hygiene

Bath time can become play time for a toddler so use that to your advantage. Give your child his or her own sponge and teach your child how to lather the soap and wash. To be fair, your child isn't going to make a good job of it at first so you will have to go over it yourself. It means bath time may take a little longer, but all the time your child thinks he or she is playing, actually learning is going on. From about 18 months a toddler can learn to rinse his or her hands properly under a tap and soon after your toddler will start to learn how to wash. Always remember that your child will do as you do before ever doing as you say, so set a good example and show your child how you do it so that he or she can copy.

Teach your child early on the difference between hot and cold taps but don't ever leave your child unattended as, although a toddler should be able to support him- or herself in a bath, your child could easily slip and fall under the water or may reach for a hot tap and be scalded.

By now your toddler is likely to have a good head of hair that will need regular washing. Most don't take to this too kindly – in fact I hated it so much I can still remember having my hair washed and the struggle that ensued as a young child even now! It's one of the reasons that throughout my childhood, I had very short hair. My mum said she just got fed up with the fuss at bath time. If your child is like me then actually keeping hair short is not a bad idea. While the hair is still soapy try moulding it into a Mohican or other shape – it can induce hoots of giggles and make a child forget how much they hate hair washing! Most kids prefer to hold their heads backwards rather than forwards to avoid getting soap and water in their eyes, but let them choose and maybe even let them hold the showerhead or fill the jug that you are using to rinse their hair. You can also try folding a flannel and allowing them to hold it over their eyes while you rinse. Use a specially formulated baby shampoo which will cause less stinging if it should get in the eyes, and always praise good behaviour. They will soon learn.

It can be easy when we are busy to sometimes feel the need to rush bath time but in my experience, this is usually a false economy. A resistant child will take so much longer to get through bath time and then is more likely to be fractious just when you want him or her to settle down for bedtime. Easy to say I know, but if you can stay calm and relaxed through bath time, so will your child.

Try to get your child used to having his or her nails cut early on. Long nails will only scratch you, friends or your child, so short nails are the name of the game. I chose to use nail clippers as I found these easier and safer but blunt-ended scissors will do the job just as well.

By the age of three, your child is likely to start to understand explanations so tell him or her why it is important to wash, and especially why we should wash hands after we have been to the toilet and before we eat.

5

Toileting

Children are different and that goes for bladder and bowel control as much as anything else. Most kids will be able to control their bowels before they can control their bladders and, as a general rule, by the age of one most kids have stopped having a poo in their nappies at night. By the age of two, some children will be dry by day but this is still quite early. By the age of three, most children will be mostly dry during the day with the occasional accident and by four they should be reliably dry during the day.

Potty training

I know it is easy to get very hung up on toilet training but it really isn't a race and just like everything else, children will develop at different rates. Boys are often slower to potty train than girls and while some kids cotton on to the idea within a few days, others will take several months. As a rough guide, most toddlers will be mostly dry by day at three years and by night at four, but one in six kids is still wetting the bed when they start school.

I know it can be difficult but try not to be too regimented about training – just because one child is out of nappies at three doesn't mean the next one will be. I'm a great believer in taking the lead from them. A child that is ready to toilet train will start to show an interest in others going to the toilet and may start to play with the potty.

When the time is right, make sure that the potty is always readily to hand and dress your child in easy to remove clothes – you may not be given much warning! Trainer pants rather than nappies make the job a lot easier. Success should always be praised, but never chastise an accident – simply clear it up with the minimum fuss and try again later.

If your child is showing no signs of improving you may have started training too early and, rather than frustrate everyone, you will be better to put the potty away again for a month or so and start again later. I also cheated slightly and waited for the summer months when there are fewer layers and, practically, it is easier to start potty training. I would never advocate delaying training in a child who is clearly indicating they would like to start but if you aren't getting any clues from your little one you could make your life easier by starting in the summer!

Once potty training is established you will want to move on to encouraging your child to use the toilet. A child's trainer seat that clips on to the toilet will make your child feel more secure. Some kids even use this straight away and bypass the potty. You will also want a step, which should be kept in the toilet to help your child get on to the toilet but also resting their feet on that step will put them in a better position to open their bowels.

It's a good idea to get children into the habit of washing their hands after going to the toilet as early as possible. Make sure you have fun soap dispensers in the bathroom and lavatory which kids will want to use.

Bedwetting

Bedwetting, or nocturnal enuresis, is a common childhood problem. Generally we expect kids to be dry at night by the age of five but in fact 1 in 6 six-year-olds and around 1 in 20 eleven-year-olds still regularly wet the bed, with boys being affected more often than girls. Most toddlers, even those who are ahead of themselves and generally dry at night, will occasionally wet the bed.

I sometimes think that we, the medical profession, don't take bedwetting in older children seriously enough. We churn out statistics and reassurance that most will simply grow out of it given time (only 1 in a 100 adults continue to have difficulties), but that's easy to say when it's not our washing machines that are constantly in overdrive.

To be fair, under the age of seven, it probably is best to wait and see but the child who has been dry at night and then starts wetting again could be stressed or anxious about something.

My toddler seems to be constantly 'playing with himself'. Is this a problem?

Toddlers 'play with themselves' for the same reason adults do – it feels nice! Not all adults masturbate and similarly not all young children show an interest in their private parts but many do and it's normal. Children under three are constantly exploring with their fingers and fiddling with parts of their bodies, whether it's their toes or their genitals – it is all part of growing up. It's often most noticeable when they come out of nappies and have the new-found freedom of pants but as parents it is best not to make a big issue of it. Constantly berating them for having their hands down their pants is unlikely to work and at worst could leave them with hang-ups in later life and feelings of guilt over experiencing physical pleasure. Toddlers are easily distracted and we use this to our advantage all the time when trying to cajole them into doing or not doing something we want – managing the masturbating child is no different. Keeping a favourite soft toy in your handbag may be all you need to save your blushes in front of your mother-in-law!

Parents often ask me if masturbation could be a sign of exposure to inappropriate sexual behaviour and in an older child explicit sexual role play can be a worrying sign, but toddlers don't have the mental maturity to act in this way. A small child who has been sexually abused is more likely to become withdrawn and revert to wetting him- or herself than to react by masturbating.

6

Sleeping

All children are different so I don't want to be too regimented about sleeping patterns but I think it is useful to have a guide on how much sleep children will need as they grow. Below are some average figures, but remember they are averages and not only does every child differ but also individual children will vary from day to day. You will notice that when they are having a growth spurt or after particularly active days their sleep requirements may change considerably.

- At 12 months your child is likely to need about two and a half hours sleep during the day and 11 hours at night.
- At two years he or she is likely to need one and a half hours in the day and 11 hours at night.
- At three years, 45 minutes in the day and 11 to 12 hours at night is needed.
- At four years your child should no longer need a routine daytime sleep but will need 11 to 12 hours at night.

The bedtime routine

You may feel like the words *routine* and *toddler* don't belong in the same sentence together and I do empathize, but it is worth trying to formulate a pattern so that your child knows he or she is winding down to bedtime. I always found bath time was a great way to start the process. I will concede that it didn't always go to plan and there were times where very excitable bouts of giggles over bubbles were anything but calming, but at least the kids knew that bedtime was imminent. There were times after a busy day at work when I was sorely tempted to skip bath time but I often paid the price. It's surprising how kids, as much as they may fight it at times, actually like routine. In our house bath time was followed by some time downstairs as a family and then story time in a more dimly lit room, before a kiss goodnight and 'tucking in'.

I always used to leave a lamp on at night and the bedroom door slightly ajar. As children grow their imaginations do too and it is natural for toddlers to show a fear of the dark. Even now I have vivid memories of seeing gremlins in the patterns of my bedroom curtains when I was a kid! I also remember pretending to be scared of the dark so that I could go and spend some more time downstairs with mum and dad and I'm sure my kids did the same. If children come downstairs it is important to reassure them and calmly take them back upstairs rather than let them learn that they can get away with it. If you haven't had much time with them during the day it can be tempting to give in, but consistency is the name of the game and if you can achieve that, your life will be so much easier in the long run.

What temperature should the bedroom be?

If children are too hot or too cold they will not sleep as well so aim for a temperature between 16 and 20 degrees centigrade.

Getting your baby out of the cot and into a bed

When to move your child from a cot into a bed is very much a personal decision – some choose to do it as early as 18 months while others keep their babies in cots well into their third year. To a certain extent the timing is often dictated by the individual child and circumstance. If your toddler has mastered escaping from the cot it is probably safer to get on with it sooner rather than later and if baby number two is imminent, it's a good idea to make the move several weeks before the new arrival to avoid any problems with sibling rivalry.

Some children will take to a new bed literally overnight (especially those with older siblings who see it as a milestone in catching up) but others find it more of an ordeal. To ease the way, try to involve them in the decision making. Take them along to choose the bed and let them help you make it up. Try to keep the bed in the same place in the room and allow your child to take his or her cot blanket and toys to bed. If you don't already have one, a night-light will make the room less scary. Inevitably, your child may take the new-found freedom as an opportunity to join you downstairs at regular intervals. Simply guide your child back upstairs without lots of cuddles and he or she will soon get the message.

Nightmares and night terrors

Most kids will have nightmares from time to time and some will get night terrors. Nightmares occur in a lighter sleep so can be recollected and older children will be able to tell you what they have been dreaming about. They are particularly common in children between the age of three and six, but if they are frequent it could be a sign that something is really worrying your child, so take time during the day to talk to him or her and find out if there are any deep-seated anxieties. Most kids grow out of nightmares and, while we may still have the occasional nightmare even into adulthood, they are rarely an ongoing problem.

Night terrors occur in a deeper sleep and the child may appear very distressed. The child may scream and thrash about and may even have his or her eyes open but not be awake. Night terrors can last for anything up to 15 minutes and because they occur in such deep sleep, the child will have no recollection of them. They can occur more than once a night. Like nightmares, children usually grow out of them. If they occur it is important to stay as calm as you can and reassure your child that you are there and that everything is OK. Try not to wake your child in the middle of a night terror as he or she will be in a very deep sleep and waking suddenly could cause more disorientation and distress. In some children a night terror will occur at the same time every night and if this is the case, you could try waking them quarter of an hour before an anticipated night terror and taking them to the toilet to break the cycle.

Sleepwalking

Like night terrors, sleepwalking occurs in deep sleep so if your child sleepwalks, the same rules apply. Your child may have his or her eyes open but will not be aware of you and may even walk straight into you. Simply guide your child back to bed and only wake him or her when settled back into bed. If your child is a regular sleep-walker, you will need to take measures to ensure his or her safety, such as moving furniture and installing a stair gate. Regular sleep-walking can also be due to underlying anxiety so take some time to talk to your child during the day about anything that may be on his or her mind.

7

Teething

Your child's first tooth is a memorable milestone that is likely to appear at around six months for most children; although, I have met babies who were born with a tooth already in place and some kids who still have no teeth on their first birthdays.

Normal development

The first teeth to erupt are usually the lower two front teeth (the incisors) and, if you are on the lookout, you will notice a pale swelling in the jaw just before the teeth break through. The next teeth to appear will be the upper incisors, followed by the teeth either side of these (the lateral incisors), and then the lower lateral incisors. Next come the first molars in the upper jaw. These are the bigger teeth towards the back of the jaw and they are soon followed by the lower first molars at around 12–14 months. The upper canines come in around 16–18 months followed by the lower canines and then the second molars in the lower jaw. The last teeth to erupt will be the second molars in the upper jaw.

In all, there are 20 milk teeth and they should all be through by the time your child is two and a half years old.

Caring for your toddler's teeth

Baby teeth help to guide the permanent teeth, which start to appear at about six years of age so it is important to look after them well. Get into the habit of cleaning them at least twice a day – decay in milk teeth can spread to the bone beneath and affect the health of the adult teeth. It's particularly important to clean teeth after the evening meal and before bedtime to ensure that no food particles are left in the mouth overnight. As your child grows, he or she may want to hold the toothbrush and I think it's a good thing to encourage this but young children simply can't be expected to clean their teeth properly on their own, so you will need to finish the job and will probably need to supervise tooth brushing until your child is about seven years old.

I found the easiest way to clean teeth was to sit one child at a time on my lap with his or her back facing me. For fidgety children who don't keep their heads still, rest your hand on your child's head to steady him or her. Use a soft-bristled brush and a tiny smear of toothpaste up until the age of three, and a pea-sized blob of toothpaste thereafter. The toothpaste should contain fluoride but not sugar. Too much fluoride can cause fluorosis, a condition that discolours the teeth.

Teeth and diet

Healthy teeth need a diet rich in calcium and vitamin D, which your child will get from dairy produce, oily fish and eggs. Your child should also be having daily vitamin drops.

Sugar is harmful to teeth. Even tiny amounts of sugar in our diet can reduce the acidity of the mouth for half an hour at a time allowing dental decay. Wherever possible use savoury snacks and sugar-free drinks but if you are going to give sweet foods, give them all in one go. Frequent exposure to small amounts of sugar is more damaging than a single large dose.

Coping with teething

You will know when your child is teething because he or she will dribble and will want to chew constantly. The cheeks may look red and your child may be irritable. He or she may also develop nappy rash but, contrary to popular belief, teething doesn't cause a temperature or vomiting so don't dismiss these symptoms. As a general rule, the larger teeth at the back are likely to be more painful. All three of my children used a teething ring, which I kept cool in the fridge and there are a variety of sugar-free teething gels available from chemists. Chewing on chilled carrots or an unsweetened rusk can be soothing, but never leave your child unattended with food as a piece could break off and cause choking. Protect your child's delicate skin from becoming sore from dribbling by applying a barrier cream to his or her chin. If your child is in a lot of discomfort, don't be frightened to use sugar-free paracetamol liquid for pain relief.

When should I start taking my child to the dentist?

It's a good idea to start taking your child to the dentist as soon as his or her milk teeth appear. Try to make it a fun, positive experience. Even if you don't like the dentist yourself, try not to show your child and, if needs be, get your partner or a relative to go instead so that the child doesn't learn your fear. Your dentist will advise you on how regularly your toddler should have his or her teeth checked.

You can get fluoride varnish, which can be applied to milk and adult teeth from the age of three. The varnish strengthens the enamel and can be applied twice a year.

What about dummies?

Dummies, it seems, are like Marmite – you love them or hate them. I chose not to use them with my children but I know for many mums they can be a godsend as a means of pacifying a crying or irritable child.

Much has been written about the overuse of dummies and dental development. Dummies won't damage your child's teeth but they can encourage an open bite, which is where the teeth move to make room for the dummy (or a thumb in thumb suckers). There won't be any permanent damage as long as your child gives up the habit by the time his or her adult teeth come through, but it can be a habit that is hard to break, which is why some mums choose not to start using a dummy at all.

If you do use a dummy, try to wean your child off it by the time he or she is starting to speak as there is some evidence that dummies can affect speech development. There is also a study suggesting that using a dummy during the day prevents the child from mimicking facial expression, which is the way babies learn about communication. The researchers noticed that children who used dummies for prolonged periods scored badly on various different measures of emotional development. This didn't apply to children given a dummy at night, presumably because kids are not trying to mimic facial expressions at night. Fascinatingly, though, the effect seems to be specific to boys. It is not clear whether this is because parents in some way compensate and encourage emotional development in other ways in girls.

It's an interesting study, which needs further investigation. I'm not about to suggest all dummies be thrown on the funeral pyre on the back of it, but it is thought provoking.

8

Travelling with toddlers

Travelling with toddlers takes forward planning so whether you are going for a day trip or a foreign holiday, you will need to think ahead and always pack extra to cover unforeseen delays. I remember, for several years I carried wet wipes with me wherever I went and never regretted it! You will probably be in the habit of packing a bag to take with you wherever you go by now. Here is my list of essentials and, as I say, always over-pack just in case:

- changing mat
- nappies
- wipes
- nappy sacks or bags to keep dirty nappies in
- nappy cream
- any medicines that your child may be taking
- toddler bowl, spoon and cup
- bib
- ready-made toddler meals
- drinks
- snacks
- a favourite toy or comforter – essential!
- hat – to protect from the sun in warm weather and the cold in winter
- a change of clothes.

Does my child need his or her own passport?

Your child will need his or her own passport. This will last for five years, even though, obviously, your child will change a lot in that time. Obtaining a passport can be quite a time-consuming process, so allow at least a couple of months for the passport to come through. You can fast track this process but at a considerable fee so it is better to think ahead. When you apply you will need to provide the completed form (available online or from post offices), two passport photos of your child, one of which must be signed by a professional who knows your child and has known you for at least two years, and proof of your child's birth, such as a birth certificate.

Do I need to pay for a seat on a plane for my toddler?

Most airlines will allow you to take a child under two for free, but that does mean you will be expected to sit your child on your lap and the cabin crew will provide you with a special seat belt to help restrain your child while the seat belt signs are lit. There have been some concerns as to how safe this is though and you may prefer to pay for a seat and take your car seat with you. If you are planning a holiday with your toddler, here are my top tips on planning ahead.

Vaccinations

Plan well ahead on this one. Your practice nurse will be able to advise you on whether your current vaccines are up to date and what you and your toddler will need depending on your destination. Some vaccines are available on the NHS as they protect against diseases that pose a significant threat to public health if they were to be brought back into the UK. These include diphtheria, polio and tetanus (given as a single booster), typhoid, cholera and hepatitis A. You may be asked to pay for other vaccines such as yellow fever, hepatitis B, tuberculosis (TB) and rabies.

Medicines

If you or your child is on prescription medication, make sure you have plenty to cover your holiday. If your prescription is likely to run out while you are away, your GP will be happy to prescribe for you early but remember it may take a day or two for that to be processed. Take a list of all prescription medication with you so that if medicines are lost you will be able to tell a local doctor what you are on. Drugs have different names in different countries so make sure you know the generic as well as the brand name. Always carry prescription medication with you in hand luggage to allow for delays or lost luggage.

Travel sickness

Lots of children suffer with travel sickness and if yours is one of them, you can try to reduce the effect by travelling while your child would usually be asleep, as travel sickness is less likely if the brain is not being stimulated by the motion of the vehicle you are travelling in. Try to avoid big meals before travelling. If you are travelling by car, try to keep the car well ventilated and avoid strong smells such as warmed food or perfumes as these can make things worse. Try playing music to distract your child but don't use toys or books to do this as this can exacerbate symptoms.

First aid kit

Of course you hope you won't need this while away but a basic first aid kit saves a lot of hassle for minor injuries and upsets. Below is a list of my first aid essentials:

- antiseptic
- simple painkillers such as paracetamol and ibuprofen
- antihistamines
- insect repellent
- rehydration sachets
- anti-diarrhoea medicine
- travel sickness pills
- a small selection of plasters and bandages.

Sunscreen

It is all too easy to reach for last year's sunscreen but check the best before date. Sunscreen becomes less effective past this date so you may think you are protecting yourself and your family when in fact the sunscreen you are applying is less effective than you think. Always buy a sunscreen that has both a high sun protection factor (SPF; at least 15 and preferably 30) and a high star rating to ensure protection from both UVA and UVB rays. Just one episode of sunburn as a child can double the risk of skin cancer as an adult, so I can't stress how important it is to take this one seriously. As a general rule, if your shadow is shorter than you then the sun is strong and it is better to keep small children out of the sun altogether.

Insurance

Even basic medical care in some countries can be very expensive so always make sure you have travel health insurance. If you are travelling within the European Union or to Iceland, Liechtenstein or Norway, you will be entitled to reduced cost or sometimes free health care if you have an up-to-date European health insurance card (EHIC). These are valid for five years and you can apply for a replacement up to six months before the expiry date. You can apply on behalf of your partner and children under the age of 16 (or 19, if in full-time education).

Jet lag

If you are travelling through time zones, try to minimize jet lag by setting your watch to your destination time as soon as you board the plane and eat and sleep as much as possible in that time zone. When you arrive at your destination make sure you get out into natural daylight to allow your brain to acclimatize as quickly as possible. It's difficult to control your toddler's body clock in the same way but at least if you arrive refreshed, you will be able to cope if your child is a little fractious as a result of the disrupted routine.

9

Vaccinations and the diseases they protect against

The vaccination schedule

If your child is registered with an NHS GP, you will automatically be sent appointments for vaccinations and I would urge you to attend those appointments as a priority. All three of my children had every vaccine offered to them and I would do the same today. You only need to meet one child with complications from one of these infections and the devastating effect these have had on the family to be convinced of the benefit of vaccination.

Your child will hopefully have already had several vaccinations in his or her first year. Below is what you can expect between now and starting school.

12–13 months

- MMR (measles, mumps and rubella)
- Hib/Men C booster (fourth dose)
- pneumococcal (PCV) vaccine (third dose)
- meningitis B (third dose).

2, 3 and 4 years

- Influenza vaccine (flu) – annual dose.

3 years and 4 months

- 4-in-1 (DTaP/IPV) pre-school booster
- MMR (second dose).

Can the vaccinations be given if my toddler has a cold at the time of the appointment?

As long as your child does not have a fever, your doctor will probably advise that you go ahead and let your child have his or her vaccinations. If in doubt speak to the surgery and they will advise you and rebook if necessary.

The vaccinations

MMR vaccine

This vaccine contains weakened versions of the viruses that cause measles, mumps and rubella. Thousands of column inches have been written about a possible link with this vaccine and autism but despite multiple research projects, no link has ever been found. Autism is, of course, a disorder of communication and socialization so it inevitably starts to present at a time when your child begins to speak and communicate, which is precisely when we give the vaccine. I am totally happy that there is no link. All three of my children had both doses of the MMR and I would do the same today.

I am often asked about the possibility of giving children the single vaccines – namely, giving the measles, mumps and rubella vaccines separately. These vaccines are not licensed here in the UK and have to be given some time apart so you simply run the risk of leaving your child exposed to these viruses for longer. The MMR can cause swollen glands for a couple of days and a measles-like rash for up to 3 days but these symptoms are not contagious.

Hib/Men C booster

Again this is an inactivated vaccine designed to boost immunity to these infections in your child's future.

Pneumococcal vaccine

This is also given as an injection and may cause a mild fever, redness or hardness at the site of injection.

Meningitis B vaccine

This is also given by injection. It is made from three proteins found on the surface of the meningitis B bacteria. It has no active ingredient so it cannot cause meningitis. It may cause a fever 24 hours after vaccination and some redness at the injection site. Your child may also be slightly irritable for a short period.

The influenza (flu) vaccine

The flu vaccine for children is given as a nasal spray rather than an injection, which is thought to be even more effective than the injection form and is obviously more acceptable to children. It is given every year because the virus that causes flu changes each year so the vaccine has to be adapted to ensure it is effective against the current year's strain. It is given to children aged two, three and four and in school years one and two.

4-in-1 vaccine

The 4-in-1 vaccine is also sometimes referred to as the DTaP/IPV vaccine. It is given as a single injection, usually into your child's thigh. It protects against diphtheria, tetanus, whooping cough (pertussis) and polio. It may cause your child to be a little irritable that evening and to develop some redness around the injection site. There is no active ingredient in the vaccine so it is safe.

The illnesses we vaccinate against

Haemophilus influenzae type B (Hib) infections

Haemophilus influenzae type B is a bacteria that can cause a number of different problems, including meningitis, pneumonia and septicaemia (blood poisoning). It causes a very serious infection – 1 in every 20 children who develop Hib meningitis don't survive and many of those who do can be left with deafness, learning disabilities and epilepsy. Hib is spread in the same way as coughs and colds but is thankfully rare in the UK since the Hib vaccination was included in the childhood vaccination programme in 1992.

Meningitis B and C infection

Meningitis is an infection of the membranes that cover the brain (the meninges). It presents with a high fever, but cold hands and feet. Children may be floppy and listless and off their food. Younger children may have a high-pitched cry and the skin may look blotchy. Older children may complain of a stiff neck or a dislike of lights. A red or deep purple rash may also develop that doesn't blanch under pressure. You can test this by rolling a glass over the rash. If it doesn't fade, it is a medical emergency and needs hospital treatment with antibiotics urgently. About a quarter of children who develop bacterial meningitis will have long-term problems such as blindness, hearing loss or learning difficulties after the infection; some will lose a limb.

Measles

Measles is a highly contagious viral infection. Symptoms usually develop ten days after the initial infection and start with cold-like symptoms. Sufferers go on to develop sore red eyes and may be sensitive to light. They can have a very high temperature (up to 40 degrees centigrade) and they develop white-greyish spots on the inside of the cheeks. These are called koplik spots. A few days later the classic pink-brown blotchy rash appears. It starts on the head or neck and spreads across the body. Sadly, there are some serious complications associated with measles including meningitis, seizures, hepatitis and blindness. There is a very rare but fatal problem that affects 1 in 25,000 people who have had measles where the brain becomes inflamed several years after the initial infection. Patients usually die within 1–2 years of diagnosis. Some live longer but, sadly, it is always ultimately fatal.

Mumps

Mumps is a viral infection causing swelling of the parotid glands, which are glands found at the side of the face just in front of the ears. Sufferers may also get a high fever and joint pains. It can also cause swelling of the testicles in boys and the ovaries in girls. Very rarely it can cause a form of meningitis.

Rubella

Rubella is another viral infection that can cause a high fever, cold-like symptoms, aching joints, swollen glands and a pink spotty rash. It is spread in the same way as coughs and colds.

If a pregnant woman contracts rubella it can have very serious consequences for the unborn baby including blindness, deafness, brain damage and heart abnormalities.

Pneumococcal infections

These infections are caused by a bacteria which can cause a wide variety of infections, the most serious being blood poisoning, pneumonia, meningitis and infections of the bones (osteomyelitis) and joints (septic arthritis).

Influenza (flu)

Influenza or flu is a viral infection, which can cause unpleasant symptoms for children including a high fever, muscle aches, headache, sore throat, dry cough and a stuffy nose. Symptoms may last for over a week and occasionally complications such as pneumonia or middle ear infections develop.

Diphtheria

Diphtheria is a highly contagious and potentially fatal condition caused by bacteria spread via coughs and sneezes and by contact with infected people or their clothing. Thanks to the vaccination programme it is now very rare in Britain. Symptoms include a high fever (38 degrees centigrade or more), a sore throat with a thick greyish coating at the back of the throat and problems breathing. It is usually diagnosed with a swab test and needs urgent treatment with antibiotics to prevent potential complications affecting the heart and nervous system.

Tetanus

Tetanus is caused by bacteria getting into a wound. It is a serious and potentially fatal condition but is now very rare because of the vaccination schedule. I have only ever seen one case of tetanus in my clinical career and that was when I was working in outback

Australia, where I looked after an Aboriginal man who developed tetanus after the tribal doctor had been packing his leg wound with dried camel dung.

The symptoms of tetanus include a high fever, rapid heartbeat, sweating and stiffness of the muscles of the jaw, sometimes referred to as lockjaw. There are often also painful muscle spasms elsewhere in the body. It is treated with tetanus immunoglobulin and antibiotics. Patients often need admitting to intensive care.

Whooping cough (pertussis)

Whooping cough is another highly contagious disease, which causes the characteristic 'whoop' sound as the child breathes in after coughing. The early symptoms may seem like any other cough or cold, but as the symptoms develop the cough becomes more severe and patients often cough up thick phlegm and may gag after coughing bouts, or they may even look like they have stopped breathing. The cough can last for three months and is treated with antibiotics.

Polio

Polio is now eradicated from the UK due to the very successful vaccination programme and, in fact, is likely to be eradicated globally in years to come. It is caused by a picornavirus, which is one of a group of viruses that live in the gut. In fact the virus can be detected in the stools of a polio sufferer up to six weeks after the start of the illness. Around 95 per cent of cases are mild with no symptoms or there may be a mild viral illness, but more serious cases affect the brain and spinal cord. If this happens, the individual will develop a high fever, headache and stiff neck and there may be progressive weakness or even paralysis of the limbs, and breathing difficulties if the muscles of the chest wall are involved. There is no specific treatment for polio, which is why it is so important to be vaccinated.

We are very lucky in this country to have such an effective childhood vaccination programme. I hope I have persuaded you to use it.

10

A to Z of infant ailments

Appendicitis

The appendix is a small appendage at the junction of the small and large bowel. It is about 5–10 cm long and has no known function. If it gets inflamed this is called appendicitis. It can occur at any age although is most common in teenagers, but I have seen it in toddlers so it is worth including in this chapter.

We don't really know why the inflammation happens. One theory is that faeces or food debris get stuck in the appendix, allowing bacteria to multiply. If inflammation develops, the first symptom is usually tummy pain. This often starts in the middle of the abdomen and then, over the next few hours, moves down to the bottom right-hand corner, although small children may not be able to specify where they feel the pain. Your child probably won't want to eat and will be running a fever; your child will find that lying still is less painful. He or she may feel sick and some children may also vomit.

When we examine for appendicitis, we feel over the appendix (the bottom right-hand corner of the abdomen). In someone with appendicitis this is usually very tender and the child may tense the tummy muscles to resist you, but interestingly as you let go, the pain is often worse. This is called 'rebound guarding'.

If appendicitis is diagnosed, your child will be admitted to hospital for an operation called an appendicectomy. This is usually done under keyhole surgery. If appendicitis is left, there is a risk that the appendix will burst causing what is known as peritonitis, which can be very serious.

Arthritis

Arthritis is a condition that we usually associate with older people but there is a form of arthritis known as juvenile arthritis that affects children and even toddlers. The child will present with painful swollen joints, which are stiff especially in the mornings or after periods of rest. The form that affects younger children under the age of six is more common in girls and most commonly affects the knees and ankles. The diagnosis is confirmed with blood tests, x-rays and scans. There are lots of different medicines that are used to relieve the symptoms and try to prevent progression of the disease. With modern treatments the outlook for kids with juvenile arthritis is now very good especially if the diagnosis is made early.

Asthma

Asthma is a very serious condition. It affects one in ten children and causes wheezing, coughing and shortness of breath. The symptoms are often worse at night and in the early hours of the morning. It is also a very variable condition and what triggers one child's asthma may be very different to the next. Common triggers include coughs and colds, cold damp air, exercise, animal fur, pollens, smoking, certain medicines and stress. The diagnosis is usually made on the history and examination and treatment will depend on the severity of the condition. Some kids will simply need a blue inhaler, which they use when symptoms are likely to flare. This inhaler opens the airways and alleviates the symptoms. If children are needing to use this inhaler regularly, the doctors will add in a steroid inhaler. This is to reduce inflammation in the airways. In more severe asthma, tablets are also needed.

Attention-deficit/hyperactivity disorder (ADHD)

This is a disorder characterized by inattention, hyperactivity and impulsive behaviour. We don't yet know why it happens but we do know that often it runs in families so if you have one child with this condition, any siblings are more likely to have it too.

Other risk factors include being born prematurely (before 37 weeks), having a low birth weight or being born to a mum who smoked, drank excessively or took drugs during pregnancy. It is more common in boys, and interestingly boys tend to be more hyperactive and girls are more prone to symptoms of inattention, which may be less obvious and can mean that girls are diagnosed later. All kids will occasionally behave like the human hurricane and that is normal, so if your toddler is giving you the run around day and night but can behave beautifully at nursery then that is not attention-deficit/hyperactivity disorder (ADHD). That is just a bright kid who has worked out he has mum or dad wrapped around his or her little finger! Just like autism (see below), making the diagnosis can take a frustratingly long time as it will involve several experts in different settings to ensure that the diagnosis is correct.

Managing ADHD will involve a number of different specialists and may also involve taking medicine.

Autism

Autism is a disorder of communication and social interaction and so it is something that starts to appear as the child begins to develop language and social skills, which is any time from about one year old. All kids will show the occasional autistic trait but a child with autism behaves in this way in all environments. It can be frustrating for parents concerned that their child may have autism because making the diagnosis can take a long time. The reason for this is that a child with suspected autism must be assessed by different health care professionals in different environments. It is important that this is done correctly because this is a life-long diagnosis. It is also important that the diagnosis is made as early as possible as the outlook for children is better the earlier the diagnosis. The symptoms that the professionals are looking for include:

- poor eye contact;
- lack of emotional expression;
- lack of interaction or interest in others;

- repeating words but not expanding his or her own vocabulary (this is called echolalia);
- lack of smiling, waving and clapping;
- sensitivity to noise and lights;
- dislike of certain textures in food.

If a diagnosis of autism is made your child will need help from educational psychologists, occupational therapists and speech and language therapists. Some children will also need medication. Autism is a condition with a wide spectrum and some children will develop good social skills by the time they are in school. In any event, it is encouraging that, with support, most children will be incorporated into mainstream school.

Balanitis

Balanitis is inflammation of the head of the penis, causing redness, soreness and swelling at the tip of the penis. There may also be a rash further down the penis. It can happen in babies, older boys and adults, but in young children it is most commonly associated with infrequent nappy changing. The urine contained within the nappy acts as an irritant so it is important to change nappies regularly and avoid other potential irritants such as bubble baths and soaps. It is most commonly treated by avoiding the irritants. Steroid, antibiotic and antifungal creams may also be needed. In rare cases, ultimately a child may be offered circumcision.

Bedwetting

Bedwetting is also called enuresis and is very common. To be fair it is common for children to need nappies at night until school age, but if your child has been consistently dry at night and then starts bedwetting, this could mean they are under stress, or sometimes constipation can cause added pressure on the bladder leading to bedwetting, so it is worth considering these options. The important thing is not to chastise your child – that will only add to any anxiety.

If your child consistently wets the bed at night after he or she has started school, talk to your GP as there are medicines available to help and special alarms that wake the child as soon as any moisture is detected in the bed and can be very effective.

Birthmarks

Birthmarks are areas of pigmented skin or a collection of blood vessels in the skin. They are not always present at birth and may develop within the first few months of life. There are several types:

- *Brown birthmarks*, these are also called moles and are permanent.
- *Stork marks*, these derived their name from the fact that they appear on the back of the neck and the forehead so were said to have been left by the stork after delivering the baby! These will fade and completely disappear in the first few years.
- *Mongolian blue spots*, these are found on the lower back or buttocks in darker-skinned babies and have in the past been mistaken for bruises.
- *Strawberry naevus*, this is a raised pink or red mark which may have a dimpled surface like that of a strawberry. It or they can be quite large and parents sometimes find them unsightly, particularly as they often get bigger and change colour before they disappear. Unless they are impairing vision we try not to treat them as they rarely cause any problem to the child and they will resolve by the age of five without treatment.
- *Port wine stain*, this is often a larger sometimes red or purple birthmark, which can become more raised over time. They are twice as common in girls as they are in boys. They can sometimes be part of a syndrome such as Sturge–Weber syndrome, which is associated with epilepsy, or Klippel–Trenaunay syndrome, which is associated with overgrowth of a limb, or Proteus syndrome, also associated with overgrowth of bone, skin or other tissues. These are rare syndromes and need to be managed by a specialist. Your GP may recommend that your child has specialist laser treatment to treat a port wine stain.

Most birthmarks will fade over time so your doctor will probably encourage you to watch and wait rather than jump in with
treatment.

Blepharitis

Blepharitis is inflammation of the eyelids. It usually affects both
eyelids and can be associated with eczema. It can cause redness
around the eyelids and stickiness around the eyelashes. You should
wash away any crusting with warm, previously boiled water and
clean cotton wool for each eye. You can also apply a thin layer of
Vaseline to the eyelid at night. If the redness persists you should
see your GP.

Blisters

A blister is a fluid-filled bubble of skin that most commonly occurs
following friction. If left alone the fluid will be reabsorbed by the
body and the skin left behind will flake off. Don't be tempted to
burst a blister, even with a clean needle as you increase the risk of
infection. If your child develops a blister on the foot, check his or
her shoes as ill-fitting footwear is the most likely cause. You can
buy special blister plasters from chemists to protect the area while
it heals.

Bronchiolitis

Bronchiolitis is an infection of the small airways (the bronchioles)
in babies and children under two. The condition usually starts with
a runny nose and cough so may seem just like a cold but then goes
on to be associated with a high fever, difficulty feeding and rapid
or noisy breathing. In severe cases the child may look blue around
the mouth and really struggle with breathing. This is a medical
emergency.

Bronchiolitis is caused by a virus called the respiratory syncytial
virus (RSV). It affects around one in three children in their first year,
especially during the winter. Thankfully most can be cared for at
home but about 2–3 per cent will need to be admitted to hospital.

Treatment includes keeping the air moist. A humidifier is great for this or, if you have warm radiators, put warm wet towels on them to encourage moisture into the air. Make sure you keep your child well hydrated and try to nurse your child slightly upright to make his or her breathing easier. It is important that you don't smoke around your toddler and that you use paracetamol or ibuprofen to control the fever. Saline nasal drops may also help clear the airways. In more severe cases, if your child is admitted to hospital, we may need to give extra oxygen.

You can protect your child from bronchiolitis by being vigilant about hand washing and keeping surfaces and toys clean. The virus can live outside the human body for several hours. Also try to avoid taking your toddler to see people with coughs and colds.

Cataracts

Cataracts are areas of cloudiness in the lens of the eye that mean vision becomes blurred. We tend to think of them most frequently as something that is associated with old age but some babies are born with what is called congenital cataracts and some develop them in the first six months of life – these are called infantile cataracts.

If only one eye is affected there is unlikely to be an obvious cause but when both eyes are affected (bilateral cataracts), they are more likely to run in the family. They can also be associated with rubella if the mother was affected when the baby was developing in the womb. If your health visitor or GP notices a cataract that has not been picked up earlier, he or she will refer your child to an ophthalmologist who will tell you whether surgery is needed to remove the cataract.

Chickenpox

Chickenpox is caused by the varicella-zoster virus. Most children will have had chickenpox before leaving primary school. Your child may be off colour with a fever and loss of appetite for a few days before the classic spots develop. They tend to form in clusters anywhere on the body. The spots start as small, itchy red spots, which then blister and, after a couple of days, they crust over. Chickenpox is infectious from a couple of days before the rash develops until the last spot has crusted over, which is usually about five or six days. You should keep your toddler away from pregnant women or anyone with a weakened immune system (such as people receiving chemotherapy) during this time. There is no specific treatment for chickenpox so it is a case of easing your child's symptoms with paracetamol, calamine lotion and cooling gels until he or she recovers. Unlike most viruses, chickenpox never completely clears from the body. After the infection it crawls back up the nerve endings and goes to sleep but later in life, particularly if you are very run down, it can reactivate, causing shingles.

Common cold

Children can expect to get anything between three and eight colds every year. They will develop a blocked or runny nose and sneezing. They may develop a mild fever and be off their food. Symptoms are usually at their worst after two or three days and then start to ease, although the associated cough may last for two or three weeks. The common cold is caused by a virus so will not respond to antibiotics (antibiotics only work against bacterial infections). Give your child regular paracetamol or junior ibuprofen to ease the symptoms and make sure they have plenty to drink.

Conjunctivitis

Conjunctivitis simply means inflammation (*itis*) of the white part of the eye (the conjunctiva). It can be caused by bacteria, viruses, irritants and allergies. If your doctor suspects a bacterial infection he or she may suggest antibiotic drops or ointment. I find ointment is often easier to use as it can be difficult to get drops accurately into the eyes of a moving toddler!

Constipation

As I have said many times before, children are very individual but, as a rough guide, you can expect your toddler to pass a motion once a day. The important thing is that your child shouldn't be straining to pass a motion. If your child is passing very solid motions and appears in discomfort when his or her bowels are open, you may want to add drinks of water between meals and you should look to increase the fibre in your child's diet by increasing the amount of fruit and vegetables. If this doesn't work, speak to your GP about which are the best laxatives to use in an infant. We prefer to use stool softeners or osmotic laxatives rather than stimulant laxatives. Stimulant laxatives work by pushing faeces through the system and may cause tummy pain. A stool softener or an osmotic laxative takes longer to work (two to three days) but is gentler on your child's system. If a youngster needs laxatives, I often find that they are needed for several weeks or sometimes months so be prepared to persevere and don't worry, your child won't become reliant on them.

Croup

Croup is a viral infection of the airways that develops the characteristic barking cough and harsh sound as the child breathes in – this is called stridor. Symptoms are often worse at night and usually only last a few days before improving but can last for a couple of weeks. Most young children can be looked after at home but some kids become very ill with a high fever, severe breathing difficulties and a blue tinge to their lips or become very drowsy and these children need to be admitted to hospital. Croup occurs mostly at around one year of age. Treatment is similar to that for bronchiolitis (see above) but your doctor may also give your child a dose of steroids to reduce any swelling in the throat and ease his or her breathing.

General hygiene measures such as hand washing and cleaning surfaces and toys will help prevent the spread of croup and it is important that you take your child for his or her routine vaccinations as some of the viruses we vaccinate against, such as measles, mumps, rubella, diphtheria, tetanus, whooping cough, polio and haemophilus influenzae type B, can cause croup.

Cystic fibrosis

Cystic fibrosis is an inherited condition where the lungs and digestive system get bunged up with sticky mucus. One in 2,500 babies born in the UK are affected. It is one of the conditions screened for at birth with the heel prick test. In the past children with cystic fibrosis invariably died young (often in their teens or early twenties) but with improved treatment and earlier diagnosis a baby born with cystic fibrosis today could expect to live until 50.

Treatment includes regular physiotherapy to help drain the excess mucus from the chest, antibiotics to treat infections and medicines to help clear the airways. Some patients with cystic fibrosis will also have diabetes and need insulin injections. Most people with diabetes are told to watch their calorie intake but this is not the case with cystic fibrosis. They need a diet high in calories and rich in fat and protein as they need to maintain weight so that they are strong enough to fight infection. The condition can affect the production of enzymes in the pancreas that aid digestion, so cystic fibrosis sufferers often need to take extra digestive enzymes to ensure they can extract the nutrients from their food. It is also important that anyone with cystic fibrosis has a flu jab every year.

If a child is diagnosed with cystic fibrosis, he or she may need extra salt as salt is lost through the skin with cystic fibrosis, but this is something that should be done under the supervision of cystic fibrosis specialists. Don't ever be tempted to add it yourself.

Dehydration

Dehydration occurs when your body loses more fluid than you take in. Older children will be able to tell you they are thirsty but if your child has had diarrhoea or vomiting or hasn't been taking fluids, you will need to look out for the signs of dehydration. The simplest thing to look out for is there being fewer or no wet nappies. If your child is potty trained and has that degree of independence it can be more difficult to notice so you will need to be more vigilant. Also try to look at the colour of the urine. It should be straw coloured. If it is darker you need to increase his or her fluid intake. Doctors also look for something called skin turgor. If you gently pinch the skin on the back of your child's hand it should fall back into place immediately you let go. If it looks tented for a while this could be a sign of dehydration. If you are in any doubt, get your toddler checked by a doctor, but like all things, prevention is better than cure so make sure you are on the lookout.

Diabetes mellitus

Type 1 diabetes is a condition where the body develops antibodies to its own pancreas resulting in reduced or no production of insulin. Insulin is the hormone we need to regulate blood sugar levels. Type 1 diabetes sometimes runs in families so if you have a relative with the condition you will be more aware of what to look out for. The child with undiagnosed diabetes may be losing weight and be excessively thirsty and passing urine more frequently. They may also complain of tummy pain and you may notice a sweet smell to their breath like the smell of pear drop sweets. If left undiagnosed and untreated, type 1 diabetes can lead to convulsions and coma so it is important to get these signs checked out.

Type 2 diabetes is where the individual develops a resistance to the insulin produced by the pancreas and this is usually linked to obesity. Type 2 diabetes used to be called maturity onset diabetes because it was only seen in adults but sadly because children are getting bigger, we are seeing type 2 diabetes in kids. The youngest child I have heard of with type 2 diabetes was just three years old, which is worrying.

Diarrhoea (loose stools)

An occasional loose stool is common in children but if your toddler suddenly develops persistently loose stools, he or she has diarrhoea. The most common cause is a viral infection, which typically will last five to seven days. It can also be caused by bacterial infection or by parasites spread from people around them and is why we are so keen on hygiene around young kids. Mo cases of diarrhoea can be managed at home but you should seek medical help if your child is showing signs of dehydration (see above). You should also consult your GP if you notice blood or pus in the motions or if your child has an associated high fever.

Ear infections

Ear infections are particularly common in young children. They cause ear ache, a fever and sometimes dulled hearing. Most ear infections are caused by viruses so simply need painkillers in the form of paracetamol or junior ibuprofen and plenty of fluids. The pain should subside within a few days although you may notice the hearing takes a few weeks to return to normal. Occasionally, the infection may cause the ear drum to burst. Because this releases the pressure, the pain is relieved but you will notice a discharge from the ear. A perforated drum usually heals itself. Very rarely a child may develop an infection in the bone behind the ear. This is called mastoiditis and is associated with increasing pain and fever. If you suspect this you should see your doctor straight away.

Eczema

Eczema is very common in children, particularly if other members of the family have suffered with eczema, asthma and hayfever. Typically the red scaly patches affect the face, neck, behind the ears and the creases of the elbows and knees but eczema can occur anywhere on the body. Eczema is basically a combination of dryness and inflammation in the skin. Make sure you keep your child's skin well hydrated with an emollient from your GP or pharmacist and apply the emollient with downward strokes. Avoid anything perfumed as this can dry the skin more and also any soaps, bubble baths or aqueous cream as these can also aggravate the problem. Avoid man-made fabrics if you can and stick to cotton clothing and bed linen. Try to maintain a constant room temperature, which is not too hot or too cold as both extremes can cause eczema to flare. If the skin is looking very red, you may need steroid creams from your GP. Parents are often worried about this but your GP will advise you how to use the cream and it is better that your child is comfortable. You will also need to keep his or her finger nails short to stop your child from scratching his or her skin. Fortunately for most kids, eczema does improve over time.

Encephalitis

Encephalitis is rare but very serious. It is inflammation of the brain tissue, which can be as a result of infection (usually viral) or as an immune reaction in a child's own body. It starts with a headache and high fever but may progress to confusion, drowsiness and even fits and coma. If you suspect encephalitis, you should get your child to hospital straight away. Investigations may include blood tests, a lumbar puncture and scans. If the diagnosis is confirmed your child will be admitted and probably nursed in an intensive care unit. Some children make a full recovery from encephalitis but, sadly, some have ongoing problems with deafness, epilepsy, personality changes and learning difficulties.

Encopresis (soiling)

Encopresis is the medical term for a child soiling inappropriately. Most children will be unaware initially that they have done it and may feel guilty as soon as they realize so try to hide it. The most common cause is an underlying constipation. If a child is very constipated a large stool can become stuck in the rectum acting as a blockage and more liquid stool can leak around the edge. It can also be linked to emotional stress – the birth of a new sibling for example. The important thing is to try not to show your frustration but to be patient with your toddler. Try not to make a big deal over toileting but at the same time get into the habit of getting your child to sit on the toilet for 5–10 minutes after breakfast without interrupting. If you think your child is chronically constipated, speak to your GP about laxatives.

Foreign bodies

Small children are always exploring their bodies and may place small objects in any orifice – ears, nose or vagina. When I was working in an ear, nose and throat department I met a four year old who had been to nursery on Friday as normal and it wasn't until the Sunday night that he coyly admitted to his mum that he had put a small bead in his ear. The poor chap had spent all weekend worrying that he might die but was also frightened that he would be in trouble if he confessed! As it turned out, he had pushed the bead in so deeply that we had to give him a light anaesthetic to remove it but no long-term harm was done. If a foreign body is left in place it can act as a focus of infection, causing a discharge.

Gastroenteritis

Gastroenteritis simply means inflammation of the stomach and intestines. It can cause vomiting, abdominal cramps, loss of appetite and diarrhoea. The most common cause is infection with rotavirus. Like all viruses, this won't respond to antibiotics. In fact antibiotics can make diarrhoea worse so treatment is with plenty of fluids, paracetamol for the pain and being fastidious about hygiene and hand washing to prevent spread to other members of the family. Gastroenteritis can also be caused by food poisoning, which could be due to bacteria and if this is suspected you should consult your GP who may want to send a sample of your child's stool to the laboratory for analysis. Some forms of food poisoning must be reported to the authorities and food poisoning caused by bacteria rather than viruses may require antibiotics.

Glue ear

Glue ear is common in children. It is when the middle ear becomes full of sticky fluid. It can affect hearing so the signs to look out for are the child who is constantly turning up the volume on the television or who struggles to follow conversation. It may not be that obvious though, and sometimes it can manifest as bad behaviour as the child gets frustrated but cannot express what is happening. It is most commonly associated with middle ear infections but can also be linked to being in a smoky environment or to allergies. If nothing is done, symptoms will improve within a small number of months. When I was a junior doctor we used to fit a lot of grommets. These are like tiny cotton reels that are placed across the ear drum to allow the fluid to drain. This is still sometimes done but less frequently. You can use an auto-inflation device, which you can get from your chemist to help clear the ear. Any child that is able to blow up a balloon is capable of using it. You simply block one nostril by pressing a finger on the side of the nose, place the balloon in the other nostril and blow. It is a bit like 'popping' your ears as you go up and down in a plane. If children have prolonged problems we may fit them with a hearing aid so that their speech and language development is not affected while they recover.

Haemophilia

Haemophilia is an inherited condition where the blood doesn't clot normally, meaning that the individual can bleed much more heavily even after a minor injury. Some people have a mild form of the condition but others bleed very heavily and can bleed internally and into joints and muscles. There are two main types of the condition and most sufferers are boys because of the way haemophilia is inherited. There is currently no cure so treatment is a combination of lifestyle adaptations to avoid injury wherever possible and injections of clotting factors when needed.

Heatstroke

If exposed to too much sun, children can develop heat stroke. In the early stages a child will develop heat exhaustion and symptoms include feeling weak and faint, being very thirsty and irritable with a headache and nausea. The skin may feel cool and clammy but they will be sweating and the temperature may rise to 40.5 degrees centigrade. If this goes unchecked, it will progress to heatstroke where the child becomes confused. Heart rate and breathing rate increase and ultimately the child may fit or lose consciousness. It is of course a medical emergency and if you suspect heat exhaustion or heat stroke you should seek medical help immediately. Keep the child indoors and undress him or her, place in a cool bath and give frequent sips of cool water until help arrives.

Hip dysplasia

Hip dysplasia is an abnormality of the hip that is usually present from birth such that the hip joint isn't as secure and stable as it should be. About 80 per cent of cases occur in girls and it is more common if someone else in the family has had the problem, although interestingly it is also more common in the firstborn child. It can also be more common if the baby was in the breech position (feet or bottom down) in the womb.

Hip dysplasia is checked for in the 6–8-week baby check. In particular, doctors are looking for asymmetrical skin creases in the thighs and for any clicking in the hip when it is examined.

If your GP suspected hip dysplasia, an ultrasound scan would have been arranged. In older babies (over four months) your GP may have arranged an X-ray. If hip dysplasia was confirmed, then you were probably given a special harness for your baby to wear permanently for six weeks. In children over six months or in those for whom the harness was not successful, doctors can put the hip into the correct position and then place a plaster cast around it to keep it in place for 12 weeks. Very rarely, if none of this works, your child may need an operation to loosen the tendons and strengthen the joint. It can be an ordeal going through all this but the good news is that the outlook is excellent if children are diagnosed and treatment started before six months of age.

Hydrocephalus

Hydrocephalus is also sometimes referred to as 'water on the brain'. Strictly speaking this isn't an accurate description, as the fluid isn't water but a special fluid called cerebrospinal fluid that surrounds the brain and spinal cord offering it protection and nourishment. The excess fluid can put pressure on the brain giving the child a headache and making him or her feel sick. The child may also have blurred vision and poor balance. It is treated with an operation to insert a fine tube to drain the excess fluid away.

Impetigo

Impetigo is a very common and highly contagious skin condition that often spreads rapidly around nurseries as small children spend a lot of time hugging and touching each other. Children who have impetigo will be asked to keep away from nursery and playgroup until they are better, which is usually within a week.

The condition is characterized by fluid-filled blisters that then crust over. While lesions are present, your child is contagious, so try to ensure your child uses his or her own flannels and towels. Once the sores have dried and healed, they are no longer contagious but this can take two or three weeks. Most cases will clear on their own but antibiotic cream or medicine, available from your GP on prescription, may speed the healing process.

Ingrowing toenail

Ingrowing toenails are relatively common in children and one of the most common causes is poorly fitting shoes or tight socks, so make sure you get your child properly measured for footwear to ensure that shoes aren't squeezing your child's feet. You also need to take care when cutting toenails. Don't be tempted to shape the nail but cut it straight across and don't cut it too short – you should be able to see the corner of the nail above the skin. You could also talk to your pharmacist about an astringent lotion which you can apply to the surrounding skin to toughen it up. If the skin around the edges of the nail is very red and painful, your child may need antibiotics to clear the infection.

Lactose intolerance

Typical symptoms include diarrhoea, vomiting, bloating and excess wind. If your doctor thinks your child may have a lactose intolerance or allergy he or she may suggest a special milk formula that has been fully hydrolysed. By that we mean the proteins are broken down into much smaller parts so are less allergenic. You can buy partially hydrolysed formula milk in the shops but if you suspect a problem talk to your GP who can advise on lactose intolerance and don't be tempted to opt for goat's milk formula unless specifically advised to do so by your GP as there can be crossover between sensitivity to cow's milk and goat's milk proteins. Your GP will also be able to advise you on a lactose-free diet.

Leukaemia

No one wants to even think about cancer in children but sadly a form of leukaemia called acute lymphoblastic leukaemia affects about 1 in every 2,000 children, and most cases occur between the ages of two and five. We don't know why it happens but there does seem to be a link to exposure to radiation and a chemical called benzene, which is used in manufacturing but is also found in cigarettes. Children with leukaemia look very pale, they are breathless and lack energy and may be prone to infection. Sometimes they bruise more easily. Treatment usually involves a combination of chemotherapy and radiotherapy and they may need a bone marrow transplant. The good news is that although the treatment is long and harrowing, most children will go into remission after their treatment.

Lice

One in five children have head lice at any one time and getting rid of them can be surprisingly difficult. The problem is that the lice are becoming resistant to the chemicals used in insecticide lotions, so that even if they are used properly and left on for 12 hours some of the lice often survive.

It's laborious, but in my opinion, the most effective treatment is to apply lots of conditioner and use a good old-fashioned nit comb. The process needs to be repeated every day until you are sure the scalp is clear, paying particular attention to the nape of the neck and around the ears, where the lice congregate. Given that the female louse lives 30 days, laying about three eggs a day and that each egg (or nit) will hatch in a week, it can take a long time to clear an infestation.

Alternatively, tea tree oil contains chemicals called monoterpenoids, which have an insecticide action, and some people find using the oil directly on the scalp is quite effective. Here is my favourite recipe – add 20 drops of tea tree oil and 20 drops of eucalyptus oil to 2 fl. oz (50 ml) of base oil (such as olive or sunflower oil), massage liberally into the scalp and hair at night and leave on for at least an hour. Comb through with a nit comb and shampoo thoroughly, but be prepared to repeat the process every couple of days for at least a fortnight. When it comes to getting rid of head lice, perseverance is the name of the game.

Migraine

Migraine is the most common cause of headaches in children. In young children, it is more common in boys than girls.

Migraine in children is different from that in adults in that it tends to occur on both sides of the head as opposed to one and is usually felt at the front and sides. Children may also complain of tummy pain and be sick and will invariably want to sleep. About one in five kids will have visual disturbances associated with their migraine, such as zig zag lines or blind spots. Some children will have no headache but present with just tummy pain and vomiting. This is called abdominal migraine.

Most kids with migraine will have a relative who also suffers. Common triggers include fatigue, stress, changes in the weather, loud noises, long periods in front of a computer or TV screen, too much activity or too much sun as well as some foods, such as Marmite, bananas and chocolate. Keeping a diary of your child's symptoms may help you to identify triggers (there is often more than one) so that, where possible, you can avoid them.

Treatment involves painkillers such as paracetamol and rest in a dark room.

If your child is getting frequent migraines, speak to your GP.

Mouth ulcers

Mouth ulcers are very common in children. The most common form are called aphthous ulcers. They are small, creamy white areas that appear on the tongue, gums and inside the cheeks. They can be very sore so your child may be off his or her food.

They can be linked to stress. Ulcers can also occur as a result of trauma so check your child's teeth for any rough areas.

Soothing gels are available from the chemist to put on the ulcers and liquorice has some natural ulcer-healing properties. Avoid salty or acidic foods while the ulcer is present as these will cause pain so keep to a bland diet until the ulcers have healed.

Muscular dystrophy

Muscular dystrophies are a group of inherited conditions that cause progressive wasting and weakness of the muscles. The most common form is Duchenne Muscular Dystrophy, which affects one in 3,500 boys (girls can carry the gene that causes the condition). Typically, a child will start to develop normally although they may be late to sit and walk, but usually while they are at primary school they will develop a waddling gait and may find it difficult to get up from the floor. They may use their hands to lever themselves up on their thighs. This is called the Gower manoeuvre. Sadly, there is currently no cure and life expectancy for children with Duchenne is reduced with most boys dying in their twenties. Work is currently being done looking at gene manipulation which could ultimately mean we find a cure for this terrible disease.

Nail biting

About 60 per cent of children will bite their nails. Thankfully, most grow out of it eventually but persistent nail biting can make the skin around the nail bed prone to infection. Try dipping your children's fingers in a bitter-tasting food they don't like to discourage the habit and make sure their nails are always cut short.

Nappy rash

Nappy rash is very common. It is caused by chafing or rubbing or by the sensitive skin being in contact with urine and faeces for too long, which is why it is important to check your child's nappy regularly and change it when soiled or wet and ensure the skin is clean and dry, paying special attention to all the skin creases before putting on a new nappy. If you can, let your toddler's bottom get some air from time to time too. If your toddler is prone to nappy rash you may like to use a zinc-based barrier cream to protect his or her skin. Most nappy rash problems can be managed at home but if there is severe inflammation, check with your GP as you may need a different cream to treat it.

Nosebleeds

Nosebleeds are common in young kids, especially boys, and are often caused by nose picking or dry air. Most will stop on their own but a small amount of blood can go a long way and they are often frightening to young children. Try to stay calm and apply pressure to the soft part of the nose for 10 minutes. This is a lot longer than you think so time yourself. If you release the pressure too early the bleeding is likely to start again so try to resist the temptation to let go and see how things are going. Keep your child leaning slightly forward so that blood doesn't trickle down the back of the throat. If the bleeding hasn't settled in this time you will need to seek medical help.

Paronychia

Paronychia is an infection of the skin next to a nail in what is called the nail fold. It can be very sore, red and swollen and sometimes there will be a collection of pus under the skin. They are most common in children who bite their nails (see above). They can be treated with antibiotics but sometimes the doctor will need to lance the skin to allow the pus to drain.

Phimosis

Phimosis is a condition where the foreskin is too tight to pull back over the head of the penis. This is normal in young children. In some boys the foreskin will start to move naturally after the age of two but for others it can take longer (until six or seven years old) and it should never be forced. If the tip of the penis becomes sore, this could indicate balanitis (see above).

Pneumonia

Pneumonia is an infection of the lungs. The child may shiver and have a high fever with cough and shortness of breath. You may see your child's tummy muscles moving to help him or her breathe and the nostrils flaring. In extreme cases the lips may have a blue tinge to them. If you suspect this you should call your doctor or take your child to the accident and emergency department of a hospital as he or she will probably need to be admitted for treatment.

Retinoblastoma

A retinoblastoma is a very rare form of cancer of the retina at the back of the eye. It affects children under five years old. It is why we check for the red reflex in babies. Of children who have this condition, 98 per cent will be cured if the condition is picked up early. It can be linked to a faulty gene so if someone in your family has had a retinoblastoma, your doctors may want to check your toddler's eyes more frequently than usual.

If a retinoblastoma is diagnosed, treatment may involve laser treatment or the application of heat (thermotherapy) or freezing the tumour (cryotherapy). Very rarely, if there is a large tumour, your child will need surgery to remove the eye.

Reye's syndrome

Reye's syndrome is a very rare but very serious condition that can cause liver and brain damage. It usually starts a few days after a viral infection such as flu or chickenpox but it can also be triggered by aspirin, which is why children under 16 should not be given aspirin. Symptoms include persistent vomiting, drowsiness, rapid breathing and ultimately fits. It is a medical emergency and children will need to be nursed in an intensive care unit. Most children will make a full recovery but sadly some kids will have long-term brain damage as a result.

Ringworm

Ringworm is something of a misnomer really as it has nothing to do with a worm but gets its name from the fact that the classic rash looks like a worm has burrowed under the skin causing a raised silvery red circle. It is actually caused by a fungal infection and is easily spread between children. You can treat it with an antifungal cream available from the pharmacist. Kids will often catch this from the family cat or dog. If you think this could be the case, take your pet to the vet for treatment, which will reduce any ongoing spread of the infection.

Scabies

Scabies is caused by infestation with a skin mite called *Sarcoptes scabiei*. It's a child's own allergic reaction to the mite, not the mite itself that causes the intense itching, which is why symptoms can develop as long as six weeks after initial infestation and may persist after treatment. The commonest sites to see the itchy papules and burrows are between the fingers and on the wrist. The mites only survive 36 hours off the skin so transmission from infected bedding is not as common as you think. There are several lotions available over the counter to treat scabies and these need to be left on overnight before washing off. Remember, you usually need two treatments a week apart and avoid applying after a hot bath as this can increase absorption into the bloodstream, taking it away from where it needs to work.

Scarlet fever

Scarlet fever is a bacterial infection caused by bacteria called group A streptococcus, which are found on the skin and in the throat. Scarlet fever usually follows two to five days after a throat infection or a skin infection such as impetigo (see above), although it can be as short as a day or as long as a week after such an infection. Initially, the child may develop a high fever, headache, flushed cheeks and a swollen tongue. This is then followed a couple of days later by a pink rash on the chest and abdomen, which then spreads over the rest of the body. It is very itchy and the skin feels a bit like sandpaper. It is treated with antibiotics but the infection is highly contagious, and your child will be contagious until at least 24 hours after starting treatment so you should keep him or her away from other children and anyone with a weakened immune system.

Sickle cell disease

Sickle cell disease is one of the diseases that is checked for with the heel prick test at birth. It affects mainly African, Caribbean, Middle Eastern, Asian and Eastern Mediterranean people. The condition is associated with abnormally shaped blood cells, which affects the ability of the body to transport oxygen effectively. The blood cells also don't live as long and it is difficult to reproduce blood cells quickly enough so that patients become anaemic.

If your child is diagnosed, you will be referred to a specialist team, which could include haematologists (specialists in disorders of the blood), paediatricians (specialists in children's medicine), physiotherapists and clinical psychologists.

Because the blood cells are an abnormal shape they can get clogged in the blood vessels, which is very painful. This is called a sickle cell crisis and the team looking after you will give you advice on how to avoid crises such as drinking plenty of water, taking regular exercise, eating well and avoiding triggers such as stress, extremes of temperature and high altitudes.

Squint

A squint is where the eyes don't look in the same direction. Most commonly, one eye looks in but it can also mean an eye looks out, up or down. It is normal for this to happen in children up to about 12 weeks of age but one in 20 children has a squint that persists after three months. If you notice this in your child mention it to your health visitor or take your child to your GP who will arrange for him or her to be assessed by an optometrist. A squint usually occurs because one eye is significantly stronger than the other and the optometrist will probably suggest using patches to cover your child's stronger eye for a short while each day. This will encourage your child's brain to concentrate on the messages from the squinting eye and improve the vision in that eye. Patching won't correct the appearance of the squint though and your child may need an operation at some point to straighten the eye.

Stammering

Stammering or stuttering is common in young children as they start to learn to speak, especially in boys. In fact as many as 1 in 20 kids will have a period of what we call non-fluent speech. The wiring of the brain is still developing in young children and as it matures around three-quarters of kids will grow out of a stammer. It is important not to make a big deal out of a stammer as that will cause stress, which will make it worse, but if you have concerns, then speak to your GP about referral to a speech and language therapist who will help you and your child through this.

Stye

A stye is a pus-filled swelling on the margin of the eyelid and it is caused by inflammation in a hair follicle at the base of an eyelash. Styes are most common on the lower lid and appear as a sore red lump on the lid margin. They often come to a head and burst after a few days. If your child will allow, you can soothe the area by applying clean cotton wool soaked in warm previously boiled water to the area for a few minutes every few hours. This will encourage the pus out. Sometimes a stye will also need antibiotic ointment from your GP.

Tonsillitis

Tonsillitis is caused by infection of the tonsils, which are found at the back of the throat. It can be caused by bacteria and viruses and it can be difficult to tell the difference just by looking without taking a swab test. Bacterial infections may need antibiotics, while viral infections need to be treated with simple painkillers and fluids. When I was a child we removed tonsils surgically (tonsil-lectomy) much more readily than we do today and that is because we now know that as children grow, the tonsils usually become less prominent and most children grow out of recurrent attacks of tonsillitis without the need for an operation. However, if your child is getting very frequent attacks (every other month for example) it is worth discussing with your GP who may refer you to an ear, nose and throat specialist for an opinion.

Toxocariasis

Toxocariasis is a rare infection caused by roundworm parasites, which are most commonly found in fox, dog and cat faeces. The eggs only become infectious after 10–21 days so fresh faeces are not a problem. However, the parasite can cause a cough, high fever, tummy pain and headache. Rarely infection can result in breathing difficulties, fits and visual problems. Mild cases need no treatment and will simply pass but more serious symptoms should be reported to your GP who will give medicine called anthelmintic. You can reduce the risk of your child contracting toxocariasis by routinely clearing faeces from the garden.

Undescended testicles

Testicles develop in the abdomen when little boys are growing in the womb and they are supposed to descend down into the scrotum about a month or two before birth. About 1 in 25 boys are born with one or both testicles not yet in the scrotal sac. This is something that will have been checked for. If one or both testicles were found to have not descended, your GP will probably have kept an eye on things in the hope that they would move down within the first six months of life, but if at six months they had still not descended, your GP would have referred you to a specialist to consider an operation to bring the testicle down into the scrotum. This is called an orchidopexy and is relatively straightforward. It is important it is done though as testes that stay in the abdomen may not produce healthy sperm, which could lead to fertility problems later in life and there is also a slightly increased risk of testicular cancer if the operation is not done. It is highly unlikely that your child would make it to toddlerhood without an undescended testicle being picked up but if you think that is a possibility, it is important that you get it checked out. There is a reflex called the cremasteric reflex which means that if you stroke the inner thigh, the testicle may retract back into the abdomen. This is normal and as long as the testicle is usually down in the scrotal sac, there is no need for further intervention.

Urinary tract infections (UTI)

Urinary tract infections are common in children – it is thought that 1 in 10 girls and 1 in 30 boys will have such an infection at some point in their childhood. They are more common in children who are constipated because constipation puts pressure on the bladder, which can mean it doesn't drain properly. Children may not complain of the burning sensation that we as adults notice with a urinary tract infection (UTI). Instead they may complain of tummy pain. They may have a fever and feel, or be, sick. They may start wetting again after having been dry. Your doctor can check for a UTI with a simple dip test of urine and most can be treated with a course of antibiotics by mouth. You can prevent future attacks by making sure that your child drinks plenty, avoiding constipation (see above), encouraging girls to wipe from front to back when they are wiping their bottoms and getting them to wear loose-fitting cotton underwear. Recurrent UTIs may be associated with problems with valves in the ureters (the tubes that carry urine from the kidneys into the bladder), so if your child has lots of urinary infections your GP may suggest that they have a scan to look into this.

Verrucas and warts

Verrucas and warts are caused by a viral infection in the skin, which causes overproduction of a substance called keratin – a hard protein in the upper layer of skin. This overproduction causes the roughened appearance we associate with warts and verrucas. They are contagious but not highly so, although warm, moist environments make them more contagious so children with verrucas should wear protection on their feet when walking around swimming pools and wet changing areas. The immune system will eventually get rid of warts and verrucas but it can take several months and sometimes even years. Verrucas can be removed by a chiropodist but the treatments are often quite uncomfortable and unless they are causing your child problems, you may prefer to just let nature take its course. There are several topical treatments available for warts. To get the best results, pare the wart down first with a pumice stone, apply the ointment and then cover firmly with duct tape.

Vomiting

Most children will vomit occasionally and usually it is short-lived, but, if your child develops a fever or has more persistent vomiting, it is likely to be part of an infective illness. The most important thing you can do is to keep your child well hydrated (see Dehydration). If you are in doubt and concerned that your child is becoming listless, has a high fever and won't take a feed, get him or her checked out immediately.

Alternatively, if there is no fever, the cause may be dietary (see Lactose intolerance above). Discuss this with either your health visitor or GP.

Worms

Worms are caught by inadvertently eating the eggs which then hatch in the gut. The female adult worms lay their eggs around the anus at night, which causes itching and the first you may know of your child having worms is an itchy bottom. Your child will then scratch while still half asleep and unless you are vigilant about washing your child's hands and scrubbing the nails immediately he or she gets up each morning, it is easy to see how he or she can become re-infested. The good news is that worms are easy to treat. You should give your child an anti-worm treatment containing piperazine, which is available over the counter from chemists. You may need to repeat the dose in a couple of weeks' time and, in the meantime, make sure you bath or shower your child every morning to remove any eggs from around the bottom and take extra care to ensure his or her hands are washed after every visit to the toilet and before eating.

11

Your toddler's medicine cabinet

I have always said that from the moment your child is born (or actually from the moment of your first positive pregnancy test!) you will have two words tattooed through you like a stick of rock and they are 'guilty' and 'worried'. It goes with the job description but so do some of the most wonderful experiences life can give you. Of course you can't be prepared for every eventuality but it is a good idea to have a basic medicine cabinet to cover minor ailments. Below is a list of what I would recommend you keep to hand:

- infant paracetamol – I'm not sure how I would have got through my children's first years without it!
- infant ibuprofen
- antihistamine ointment or syrup for bites
- a digital thermometer
- calamine lotion
- barrier cream for nappy areas
- saline drops for blocked noses
- children's nail scissors or nail clippers
- children's sunscreen
- child-safe insect repellent
- cotton wool balls and gauze swabs
- adhesive tape
- plasters
- bandages
- alcohol wipes and saline for cleaning wounds
- antibacterial ointment for cuts and grazes
- calamine for skin irritations
- syringe for administering medicine – you may find this easier than using a dropper or a spoon, but if your child will use it a dosage spoon or cup can be used
- tweezers for removing splinters.

12

First aid for toddlers

Of course I hope that you won't need the contents of this chapter but it's worth knowing what's in here so that you will know what to do if your child is in need of first aid help, or someone else around has a child who needs immediate treatment.

Allergic reaction

Common allergens include drugs, stings and bites, pollens and some foods, most commonly nuts, shellfish and eggs. The child may develop a blotchy rash like nettle rash, the tongue, lips and face may swell and he or she may develop wheezing and difficulty breathing. This is a medical emergency and you should call 999 immediately. Try to keep the child calm. If there is a known allergy, the child may be carrying an auto-injector pen containing adrenalin, which should be given straight away following the instructions on the packaging. If you have children's antihistamines available, give these while you wait for help.

Asthma attack

Asthma is very common and most children with a diagnosis will carry a blue inhaler. If the child should start to become wheezy, encourage him or her to keep calm and sit comfortably, leaning slightly forward to take the inhaler. If the wheezing worsens, you will need to seek medical help.

Bleeding

If a child has a significant cut and is bleeding heavily, try to elevate the part that is bleeding above the level of the heart and put pressure on the wound. If the bleeding is heavy you will need to call 999 and keep pressure on the wound until help arrives.

Broken bone

If you suspect a broken bone, try to support the area with clothing or cushions so that the bone can't move. If you can, transport the child carefully to the nearest accident and emergency department of a hospital. If not, call 999 and continue to support the injury until help arrives.

Burns

A toddler's skin is very delicate. Even a warm cup of coffee could cause a burn so if your child has been in contact with something hot, run the skin under cold water for at least ten minutes and then apply cling film to the area. If you are concerned, take your child to the accident and emergency department of a hospital where staff can dress it with special burns dressings and assess whether anything more needs to be done.

Choking

If your child appears to be choking, hold him or her face down across your lap with the head lower than the bottom, or lean your child forward across your arm and, using the heel of your hand, give five firm blows to his or her back. If this doesn't dislodge the offending object, try holding the child around the waist with his or her back to you and pull upwards and inwards just above the tummy button. You can repeat this cycle but if the symptoms are not resolving or if your child is looking blue, call 999 immediately.

Croup

Croup is worse in dry conditions so you need to make the air as steamy and humid as possible. Try boiling a kettle or running a hot bath but don't ever leave your child unattended in such an environment. You could also put hot, wet tea towels on any radiators. Try to keep your child as calm as possible but if symptoms aren't settling, seek medical advice.

Fever

All children will get a fever at some point. If your child has a fever, take layers of clothing off and give your child the recommended dose of ibuprofen or paracetamol. You could also try giving your child a tepid bath and cool fluids.

Head injury

Toddlers fall over – it is part of their job description and it is all part of the learning curve – but if they fall on to a hard or sharp object or from a height they can incur significant injuries. It is important not to leave your toddler unattended as accidents can happen in a split second. If your child has a bump, apply something cold, such as frozen vegetables wrapped in a tea towel, to the injury and comfort your child. If your child becomes drowsy or vomits get him or her to a doctor.

Seizures

If your child has a seizure, check the surrounding area, making sure that you move any furniture or objects the child could injure him- or herself on, but do not restrain the child. When the seizure has settled, remove any excess clothing if you suspect a fever fit, and

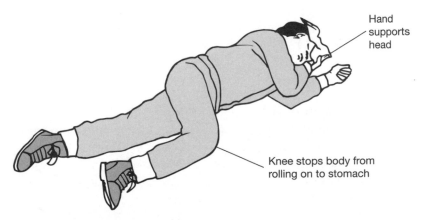

Hand supports head

Knee stops body from rolling on to stomach

Figure 1 The recovery position

give medication to reduce a fever as soon as the child is able to take it safely. If this is the first fit, seek medical advice.

Epileptic seizure If you suspect an epileptic seizure, the advice is the same. Do not try to restrain the child, and make sure you move any objects that could cause injury away from the child. After a seizure the child is likely to feel drowsy. Place your child in the recovery position (Figure 1) and stay with him or her. If this is a first seizure, it is important that you seek medical advice.

The unconscious child

If you should find your child unconscious, first of all check for breathing. If your child is breathing, support the child on his or her side with the head slightly below the bottom so that the airway stays open and call 999.

If your child is not breathing, shout for help, asking someone to call 999 while you tilt your child's head back by placing one hand on the forehead and two fingers of the other hand under your child's chin. Then pinch your child's nose, cover the mouth with yours and blow five breaths into him or her. Then push firmly with one hand into the middle of your child's chest 30 times before giving your child another two breaths and then more compressions, and keep doing this until help arrives.

13

Toddler safety

As your child becomes more and more mobile you will be on a steep learning curve when it comes to safety. When my kids and my friends' kids were growing up, we used to joke that you could tell the age of a family's children by the height of their ornaments!

The truth is that most accidents occur at home and over half of them involve children under five. The thing is, children develop quickly and they are suddenly able to reach something today that yesterday was safely out of bounds, so it is easy to be caught unawares.

Before we look at specifics, it is more important than ever now that you make sure your house is fitted with a smoke alarm and carbon monoxide alarm. Here are a few of my basic tips to keep your child's environment as safe as possible.

Kitchen and living spaces

- Always turn handles of pans away from the edge of a surface and towards the wall.
- Push jars and bottles to the back of work surfaces.
- Keep cords to kettles or other appliances at the back of the surface or preferably stick to appliances with coiling cords that naturally retract.
- Put safety catches on drawers and cupboards so that your child can't get to knives or cleaning products.
- Cover unused sockets with dummy plugs.
- Place the television and any other electrical equipment against a wall where your child cannot get to the back of it.
- Keep all ornaments high up out of reach.
- Put safety film on any glass doors.

- Keep warm drinks far away from the edge of surfaces – even a cup of coffee can give a small child a nasty burn.
- Keep pet bowls out of reach of children and clean them regularly.
- Don't use table cloths as small children may use these to pull themselves up to standing.
- If you can, keep the kitchen bin inside a cupboard secured with a safety catch.
- Remove spring loading on doors designed to make them close automatically.
- Pay strict attention to food hygiene.
- Keep cat litter trays out of reach.

Bathroom

- Use a non-slip mat in the bath and never leave your toddler unattended in the bath.
- Keep all cleaning materials, aerosols and cosmetics in wall cupboards out of reach.
- Tighten hot taps firmly so that your child is unable to open them.
- Put safety film on shower doors.

Hall and stairs

- Invest in a stair gate before you think you need one. I have seen far too many children who have fallen down the stairs because they took their parents by surprise.
- Keep the front and back doors well fastened.

Garden

- Attach childproof locks to any gates.
- Fence off any areas of water and drain a paddling pool immediately after use.
- Remove any potentially poisonous plants from your garden.

- Keep an eye on pathways and clear any moss to avoid slippery surfaces.
- Keep all garden tools and chemicals in a locked shed.
- Clear up pet excrement immediately.

Index